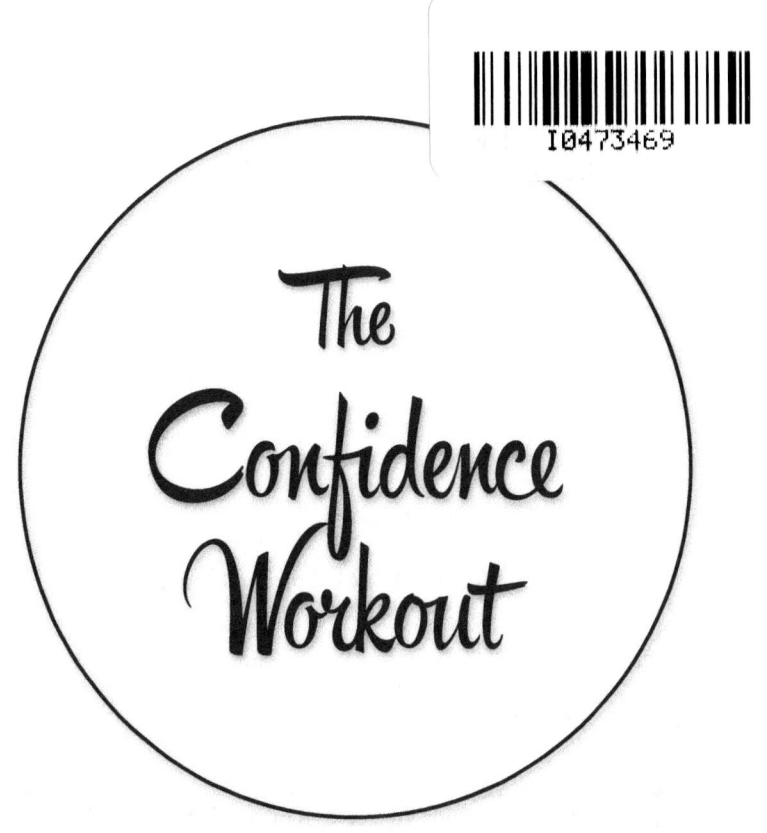

The Confidence Workout

17 surprising little ways to feel more confident at work and in your life.

Michelle Landy

The Confidence Workout

Author: Michelle Landy

Copyright © 2012 Michelle Landy

First Published in 2013 by Black Pebble Publishing
PO Box 8500
Armadale, Victoria 3143
Australia

ABN: 66790493707

The moral rights of the author have been asserted. The stories, suggestions and opinions of the author are her personal views only. The strategies, workouts and techniques in the book may not work for everyone. Due diligence, thorough research and individual guidance is recommended.

Editor: Jo McKee, www.editonline.com.au
Design: Richard Jenner, www.typeshed.com.au

ISBN: 978-0-9874119-0-7

Dedication

To my friend Lindy Alexander.

Praise for *The Confidence Workout*

'Everyone would like to be, at least a little, better at something. I don't know anybody, including myself, that wouldn't like to be a little more confident in at least one area of their life. *The Confidence Workout* is the perfect tool to help become a better, happier and more successful you. Buy this book now and feel the difference.'

W Mitchell,
Author of *It's Not What Happens To You, It's What You Do About It*

'Everyone says you need luck to succeed. Although luck helps, in my experience, I believe it is a small percentage of what helps compared to having confidence.

'People who have success and who get through adversities have the confidence to constantly turn the rudder of their lives. They have learned to control their fear and simply trust!

'Confidence is learned through practice and by surrounding yourself with people who help you discover that you have it — Michelle Landy is one of those people who can show you how to wake it up.'

Sandra Canudas
Author and Consultant

Contents

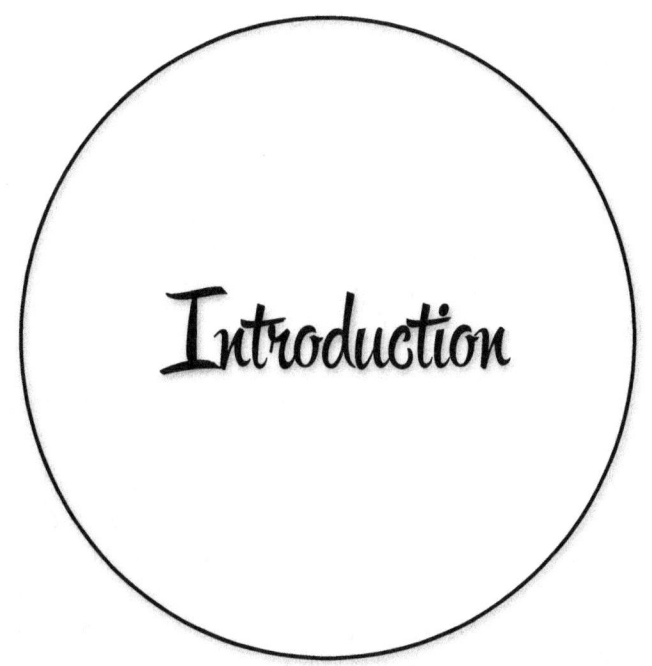

Introduction

It is the beginning of one of my workshops on confidence and everyone is taking their seats. People from so many different backgrounds have come, yet they are all here for the same reason: they want to feel more confident. That's what we all want, because it is the basis for everything we do.

Some have a specific dream and are lacking the confidence to start. Others are fed up with feeling held back at work and in their lives.

As I look around, I am always surprised that on the outside everyone looks reasonably confident. This is how we all are. We look more confident on the outside than we feel on the inside.

However, it does not matter how confident we look on the outside. What matters is how we feel on the inside. That's what we live with each day. That's what determines what we will do and how we feel.

This book is a guide to kick starting your confidence. It will show you incredibly easy ways that you can strengthen your confidence. The path to feeling confident is not as hard as you may think. There are certain things that influence confidence; there are some things you need to do more and there are other things you need to make sure you never do.

This book gives you tips and techniques to help you start doing all sorts of wonderful and exciting things — things that you may have been longing to feel confident enough to do. These techniques are what I do with my clients. I call the practice of these techniques 'workouts' because they are active, uplifting and empowering to do. Best of all, they transform how people feel and they quickly build confidence.

They have helped:

- people who once thought of themselves as shy learn to speak up with confidence and be heard;
- people who were nervous learn to present themselves with confidence and get promoted; and
- people who had hesitated for years to finally start a dream pursuit.

I've written this book because over the years I've seen what a difference it can make to people's lives to have confidence. I've seen the power of boosting confidence in my coaching clients and seen how these simple techniques transform how people feel and help people start doing more of what they love. I want you to also feel good about what you do and have the confidence to start your dreams.

These techniques work for just about any situation. They have helped my leadership students at university get the jobs they want. They have helped my coaching clients get promoted, expand businesses and start their dreams. They have helped people achieve fitness and weight goals. They work for any pursuit in which you want more confidence.

In my work helping people boost their confidence I have noticed a wonderful thing about learning to become more confident: it impacts everything in their lives. When people become more confident doing one thing, it ripples out into everything else. Much like throwing a stone in water, the ripples go out in all directions.

Let's get started. Come with me and discover the incredibly simple little things you can do that will help you activate your confident self.

Michelle

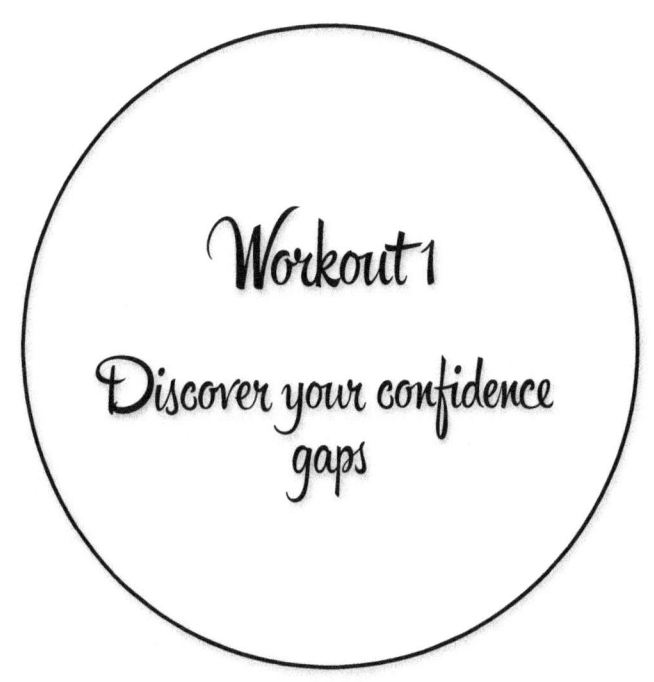

Workout 1

Discover your confidence gaps

Think about how confident you are. Could you rate it out of ten and say 'this is exactly how confident I am?'

If you are like most people you will find it hard to score. That's because your confidence depends on so many factors. One day your confidence may be high and the next day it may be low. In one area of your life you may feel like a nine and in another a two. When you do one activity it is there, but then in the next it feels like your confidence has completely disappeared.

Confidence can't be scored exactly. This is because we don't have an even amount of confidence for everything we do.

You may feel confident at home, but not at work. You may feel confident with friends, but not with new people. You may be confident with outdoor activities, but not with indoor ones.

Most people will have gaps in their confidence. Depending on what you have been exposed to, your confidence will have grown in uneven ways.

Each of us has different gaps because we all have a different history. We have been brought up in varied ways; each in a unique environment exposed to certain elements and learning to become familiar and comfortable doing particular things.

If you are doing something now in your life that you have not previously been exposed to, don't be surprised if you find you have a gap in confidence.

I was born on a farm and grew up with high levels of confidence in nature, handling animals and coping on my own. This served me well in that environment, but as soon as I moved to the city some gaps in confidence, such as comfort in using public transport, soon appeared.

These gaps are normal and to be expected. Much like weak muscles, our confidence is weak from lack of exposure, lack of practice and lack of opportunity.

A gap in confidence is not a big deal if you just think of it as weak through lack of use. Remind yourself that your confidence is underdeveloped, not broken or permanently damaged. It just needs some strengthening.

You can strengthen your confidence. Much like how you would strengthen a muscle, you strengthen your confidence through exposure, repetition and incremental immersion. You close the gaps through using, doing and immersing. But most of us don't do this. We tend to avoid doing the things we lack confidence to do.

The trouble is, the more you avoid doing the things that you don't feel confident doing, the further you weaken your confidence in those areas. What we don't use we lose. And if we are not careful, what started as a minor weakness can become a major block.

To strengthen my confidence in using public transport, I needed to actually start using it. I had to remind myself my confidence was weak in this area and not expect to be able to handle the whole network in one hit. I had to strengthen my confidence gradually, in easy ways and without pressure.

I imagine you, too, have gaps in your confidence. Don't try to become confident at everything all at once. Your aim is not to become confident at everything anyway. It is just to be confident at what matters to you.

Often the best areas to strengthen first are the things that cause you stress because you don't have confidence doing them. For example, if you have to chair a meeting regularly at work, and this causes you stress, then this would be something worth becoming confident doing because you are going to be doing it often.

Choose an area where you have a gap in confidence that you would like to strengthen. Instead of avoiding this activity because you don't have confidence, start doing it to strengthen your confidence.

Start in a way that is easy for you. Just like working your muscles, start on the easy weights with just a few repetitions so you don't overextend yourself. Then once you can comfortably cope with that, you can slowly increase what you expect and what you attempt to do.

Ask yourself this: in what situations do you want to feel more confident?

When you are being ...

- formal?
- professional?
- casual?

When you are ...

- alone?
- around popular people?
- the centre of attention?

When you have to ...

- stand out?
- talk about yourself?
- promote yourself?

When you are ...

- in the country?
- in the city?
- in a new place?

When you feel …

- less qualified?
- not pretty enough?
- not good enough?

When you are talking to …

- the opposite sex?
- younger people?
- older people?

When you are with …

- famous people?
- successful people?
- rich people?

When you …

- have to speak up?
- share your feelings?
- contribute your opinions?

When you are …

- doing physical things?
- using your intellect?
- handling emotional situations?

Ask yourself:

What gap in confidence is most impacting your life?

What gap in confidence would you most like to fill?

Remind yourself that your confidence is underdeveloped, not broken or permanently damaged. It just needs strengthening.

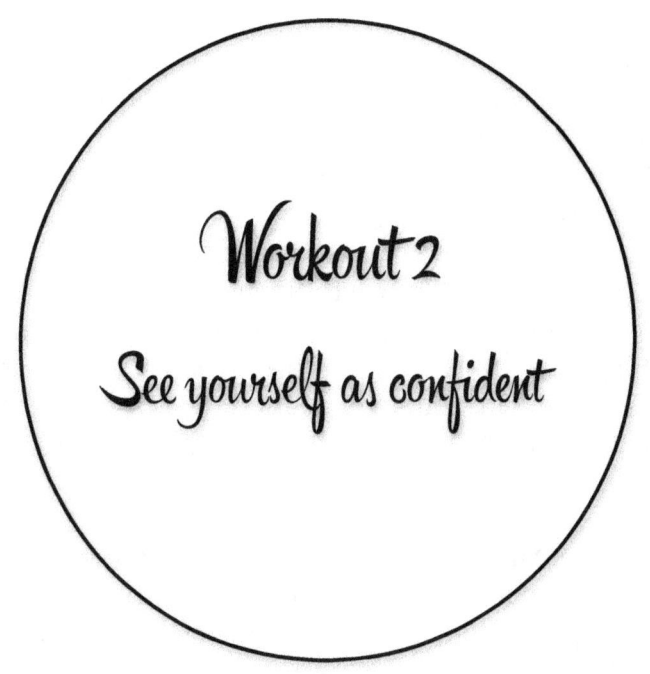

Workout 2

See yourself as confident

To become confident you have to first believe it is possible for you to be confident. This may sound strange, but many people carry limiting beliefs about themselves and about how confident they can actually be.

Many people block themselves from feeling confident by how they define themselves. They too readily label themselves as 'shy' or 'not confident', not realising that how they see themselves impacts how confident they will feel.

If you can't first see yourself as feeling confident it is virtually impossible to be confident. Your image of your confidence is the foundation and if your foundation is not right, that's what you have to rebuild first.

We accumulate our confidence-image through our experiences and how we were raised. Many things such as our past experience and past mistakes can negatively influence our image of our confidence. Other people can also greatly influence it.

If you struggle to see yourself as someone who can be confident, you may have had others telling you that you were not confident when you were a child. Because you were young, you believed it. If you had people put you down and never build you back up you may have formed mistaken conclusions about yourself. Or, if your parents didn't see themselves as confident, you may have unconsciously caught their limiting self-image and taken it on for yourself.

No matter how you came by any limiting beliefs you may have about your own confidence, what matters now is changing them. Despite what has happened to you and despite what others may or may not have said or done, being confident from today forward is a choice. It is your choice now. And the first choice is to stop letting your history and past perception of yourself define you.

Imagine you could drop your history completely. Yes, that's right. Imagine you have no history at all; that when you woke up this morning, you could no longer remember how confident you were, are or were meant to be. Nor how confident you think you should be. Can you imagine just how infinite the possibilities would be?

Confidence is not something we are stamped with once in our lives and then defined by for the rest of our lives. We can change how confident we are.

Just because you weren't confident at eight years of age does not mean you can't be now. And just because you weren't confident yesterday when you stood up and did that presentation at work, or you went to that social gathering, does not mean you can't be today.

From today, commit to defining yourself as being confident. Do not worry about your actions. Do not worry if you act in shy ways and feel nervous. Regardless of what you do, define yourself as confident.

Most people try to change their actions, but that is not the place to begin. It is your image of yourself that needs to change first. Once you see yourself as confident, it is easier to act in confident ways.

Confidence is not something that is in limited supply, nor is it only available to the lucky few. Everyone can feel its magic energy. After all, confidence was woven into our spirit at birth. It is what helped you learn to move, crawl and then walk, despite how difficult these tasks were to learn.

Your innate confidence kept you going. When you fell over, did you stop to think 'Am I confident enough to keep going?' or think 'I am too shy to keep trying?' Thankfully you had not yet formed a limiting image of yourself. You just kept going, all the time believing you would get there.

To rebuild a more positive image of your confidence, commit to never again saying 'I'm not confident.' Even in those moments when you don't feel confident, replace your thoughts with something more empowering. Say to yourself an empowering statement such as, 'I am willing to be confident' or 'Every day I am learning to be more confident.' And then notice how much better this makes you feel.

Affirmations of positive intent are a wonderful way to rebuild your self-image. Affirmative statements such as:

I am choosing to be confident today.
My past confidence does not define my future confidence.
Confidence is always in me.
I can access confidence whenever I need it.
I am worthy of feeling confident.
Confidence is for everyone.

Write out some affirmations of your own that will nurture and nourish your sense of confidence. You can be confident. It starts by changing how you see yourself and beginning to see that confidence is possible for you.

Ask yourself:

How have you been seeing yourself?

What image of yourself would help you feel confident?

Imagine you could drop your history completely. Imagine that you woke up and could no longer remember how confident you were, are or were meant to be.

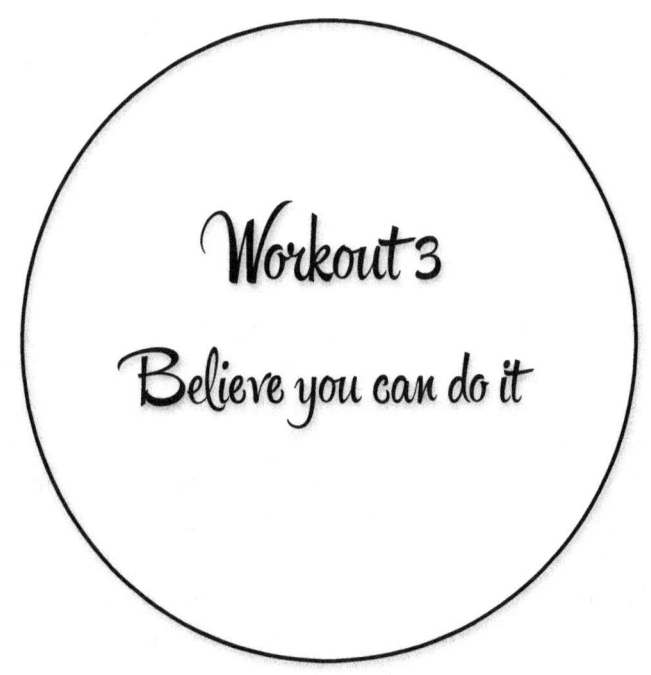

Workout 3

Believe you can do it

It does not matter how capable you are of doing something. If you don't believe it is possible to do, you won't be able to do it. Believing that something is possible is the basis of confident action. Not only does it determine what you will attempt, it also influences how you attempt it.

Jenny, a participant at one of my workshops, told me she had always wanted to have dancing lessons in Buenos Aires. She had seen a dance show on television when she was eleven years old and the idea had remained with her ever since. As she continued to talk, however, she started closing the door of possibility on herself saying, 'Oh it's just a crazy idea though. It is impossible. Someone like me would never be able to do such a thing.'

Sometimes we close the door of possibility before we fully try something. We are capable of doing something, but our lack of belief sabotages our ability and our confidence to take proper action. Our attempts become half-hearted or, even worse, we may not try at all.

Our lack of belief can exist on many levels. It can be a lack of belief in our capacity and ability. Or it can be a lack of belief in the pursuit itself; in how hard we think it is to do and how possible we think it is to achieve.

When I was in my last year of university one of my professors handed me ten coins and said, 'See if you can stack these on your elbow, flick your arm and then catch them all with the same hand.'

I didn't think it was possible and hesitantly said, 'I'll try.' Sure enough the coins went everywhere. He collected them and placed them all on his elbow. Then, to my surprise, he caught them all in one swift move.

Seeing him do it suddenly made me believe I could do it. My self-belief awakened because now I knew it could be done. 'After all,' I thought to myself, 'if he can do it, surely I can too.'

I stood up with focus and determination, stacked the coins and this time caught all ten coins.

When our belief changes, our actions change. It's not magic. It's just simple cause and effect. When we believe something is possible, we act in ways that are more likely to make it possible. Our actions are more focused and we are more determined.

Many of the things we want to do are not as hard to do as we think. Sometimes it is just how we perceive them that make them hard. Mostly this happens when we have wanted to do something for a long time and the idea has lingered too long without us taking action. Then the pursuit can feel more elusive and seemingly harder to do than it actually is in reality.

To take confident action you have to see your pursuit as something achievable and possible for you to do. If you look back over your life you will realise you have done many things that were hard, yet because you believed they were possible, they were possible for you.

Give your confidence a chance by changing how you see your pursuit. See your pursuit as a little less extraordinary to do. Take away the 'wow' factor and make it feel more ordinary to achieve. Not ordinary 'boring', but an ordinary that makes you feel like you can do it. Ordinary because ordinary will get you started.

Try this. Think about something you want to be able to pursue with confidence. Then before you even take the first step towards it, make sure you have opened the door of possibility for yourself. Make sure you start feeling like it is possible and achievable.

Do everything you can to make your pursuit feel possible. Find others who have done something similar as this can make you feel like it is more possible for you.

Spend time with ordinary people who do extraordinary things and let their sense of possibility rub off on you. Research what you want to do. Knowledge often makes things feel more possible as it helps us establish a plan. Work out what part you will need help doing and let yourself get that help; notice how suddenly it feels more possible once you know that you don't have to do everything on your own.

To take confident action you need to take the 'big deal' factor out of what you want to do and make it feel possible for you to achieve. Even if your dream pursuit is a big deal to other people, don't make it one for yourself.

Ask yourself:

How has your lack of belief impacted the actions you take?

How could you make your pursuit feel more ordinary?

Take away the 'wow' factor and make your dream feel ordinary. Not ordinary 'boring', but an ordinary that makes you feel like you can do it.

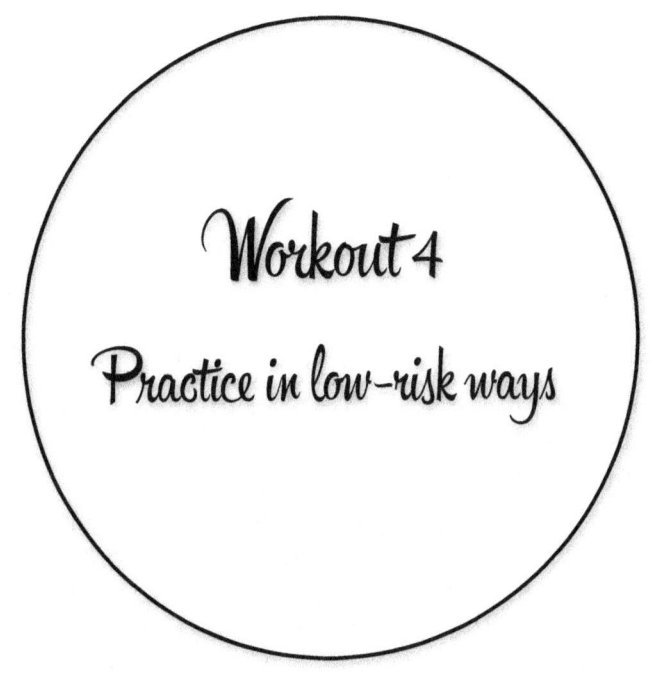

Workout 4

Practice in low-risk ways

Confidence is not something you should try to develop suddenly and all at once. It takes gradual exposure and gradual growth. If you try to rush you actually can damage your confidence rather than boost it. Sometimes we forget this and put ourselves in situations that are out of our depth — beyond our confidence experience — too soon and then end up sabotaging our confidence instead of boosting it.

When I help people learn to speak up with more confidence, I often have to remind them not to rush out and practice their new assertiveness skills immediately on their boss. After years of not speaking up, when they finally do, they risk going straight into advanced situations without first gaining some practice in speaking up in situations that have no ramifications or with easier people.

We are all at risk of doing this. When we learn any new skill, our enthusiasm to get started can make us take action too quickly, without any consideration for what might be the best action to take or the right place to start. Sometimes we mistakenly take our newfound skills straight into high-risk situations without any experience. We forget that although our enthusiasm is high, our confidence is still fragile and that it doesn't take much for us to give up.

If you leap straight into high-risk situations and get out of your depth you may never want to try again. If something goes wrong you may be at risk of blurting out that 'dream-killing' vow of 'I'm never doing that again' and completely eroding your confidence in what you are doing.

You need to make sure that you first practice in low-risk ways and with low-risk people. That way you build your confidence, not just your skill. Instead of rushing out and tackling the high mountain straight away, try to find opportunities to practice in the smaller hills first.

Confidence grows when we give ourselves opportunities to practice without risk. To build your confidence in what you are doing find low-risk ways to practice. Practice with low risk people; easy people and people whom you find less reactive, less judgemental and less intimidating.

Practice in low risk situations too. If you want to stand up to your boss and achieve an effective outcome, then don't start there. Start by speaking up generally in your everyday life more first. It's the same voice you have to find; only you are using it in an easier arena.

Make sure you are incremental in your approach. Move from easy to hard, from low-risk to high-risk situations. You didn't learn to drive your car in the middle of a busy freeway. If you are like most people you first practiced on quiet back streets where the consequences of any mistakes were less. Then you progressed to busier places and more difficult environments.

To ensure your confidence expands at the same time as your skills expand, you also need to do things progressively. Let the order build on itself in a logical way. Babies learn to crawl before they walk and they learn to walk before they run. It's progressive. It's sequential.

Make a plan as to how you will practice. Don't let it just be any old practice, but instead design practice opportunities that will expand your confidence gradually and steadily without putting it at risk. Practice in easy ways first. Then, once you have gained some confidence, you can step out into broader and more difficult situations knowing you have the confidence to cope.

My client Jessica wanted to become more confident eating on her own in restaurants. She travelled extensively for work and didn't want to feel restricted to room service. Yet for her, dining in a restaurant alone was a big leap. It was beyond her experience and her confidence. Instead of leaping she needed a plan to gradually expand her confidence.

She started in non-formal environments like coffee shops so she didn't feel pressure and judgement. She took a book to her first restaurant so that her focus was not on being alone. She sat at a side table so she didn't feel like everyone was looking at her.

Every day Jessica changed one element. Every day she stretched her confidence incrementally and progressively towards her end goal of eating alone in a restaurant. By starting in low-risk ways and gradually stretching her confidence, it wasn't long before she was regularly eating in restaurants on her own. And most importantly, feeling confident doing it.

Remind yourself that achieving confidence is very different to achieving a goal. You need to do things that expand your confidence, not just get you to the goal. Your aim is not to just be able to do something. It is to feel good when you do it.

Ask yourself:

Where can you best practice your skills so your confidence is nurtured?

How can you increase the difficulty of what you do gradually?

Instead of rushing out and tackling the high mountain, find opportunities to practice in the smaller hills first.

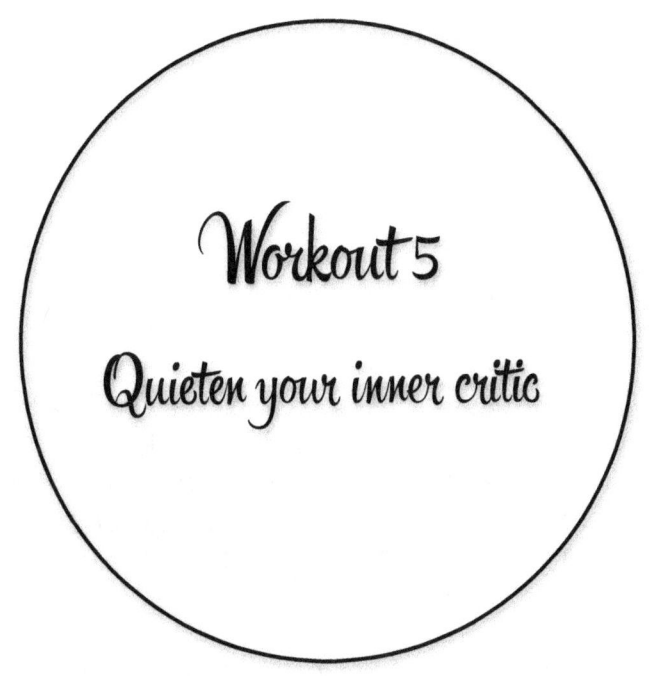

Workout 5

Quieten your inner critic

Each of us has an inner critic. You know, that part of you that endlessly judges and criticizes what you do and how you do it. Most of us know our inner critic well because it is constantly with us and has much to say. To feel confident we need to understand our inner critic and respond to it in ways that quieten it and subdue its impact.

Sometimes it can feel like our inner critic sits there waiting to lash out; its comments are repetitive, sometimes predictable and almost always crippling to our confidence.

Your inner critic may at times be harsh and cruel and act like the enemy, but its source is fear rather than hate. It is the part of you that worries about what others think, worries about not succeeding and worries about survival.

When it roars, it is the voice of fear calling out BEWARE. Beware you don't make a fool of yourself. Beware you are not wasting your time. Beware you can keep up with the group. But it does not stop at 'beware'. Instead of caution, it can start to attack.

Instead of guiding you forward highlighting its concerns, it lashes out. Instead of protection, all we hear is judgement, berating and harsh criticism. And if you are not careful, you might let your inner critic erode your confidence, making you feel like giving up.

My friend Kate had always wanted to learn to play the guitar and finally started taking lessons. Yet after just a few weeks she was already succumbing to her inner critic and considered giving up.

Every time she played, her inner critic lashed out in full swing with comments such as, 'You're too slow. You'll never be able to play well. You might as well give up.'

Her inner critic was strong and Kate was at risk of letting the harsh words erode her confidence and stop her completely. But she didn't. She learnt how to kept playing despite the words in her head.

This is what we must do. When your inner critic lashes out, do not let your confidence crumble beneath its reckless comments. It's time to rein your inner critic in. It's time to stop its crushing impact and learn to become less influenced by what it says.

When your inner critic lashes out, don't accept what it blurts out. Sometimes we make one mistake and our inner critic lashes out and blankets everything with judgement. You may play one chord the wrong way and your inner critic can make you feel like you have played the whole song incorrectly.

Don't let your inner critic lash out unrestrained. Ask your inner critic to be specific. Make it contain its judgements to exact examples, so you don't feel overwhelmed by what it says.

If there is one part of the song that you strum badly on your guitar, don't accept that voice that says 'you can't play this song' or worse still 'you can't play at all.' Make your critical voice articulate itself. Make it focus and comment only on the specific mistake. Make it say 'you can't do that one chord transition very smoothly.'

One chord does not overwhelm us. One chord does not crush our confidence. When we force our inner critic to focus its comments, its voice becomes less harsh and we can hold our confidence in place.

When your inner critic rises up, speak back. Don't stay quiet and just accept its comments. If you are learning the guitar and you hear your critic start niggling away with comments like, 'you are useless' or 'you are slow', then answer with kindness and compassion for yourself. Say:
- of course I am not very good; I am a beginner
- of course I am not competent; I am a beginner
- of course I am learning what to do; I am a beginner

If your inner critic won't be quietened and speaks louder and stronger, do not stop to give it attention. Hear it and then keep playing your guitar regardless of what it says. When it bombards you with judgement, keep going.

No matter how bad your performance, keep strumming.

No matter what crazy put-downs it blasts you with, keep playing.

No matter what comments your inner critic has to say, keep going.

Don't stop to listen to your inner critic. Just keep going, because nothing silences your critic more than action.

Ask yourself:

When does your inner critic lash out?

What will you do when your inner critic speaks?

Don't stop to listen to your inner critic. Just keep going, because nothing silences your critic more than action.

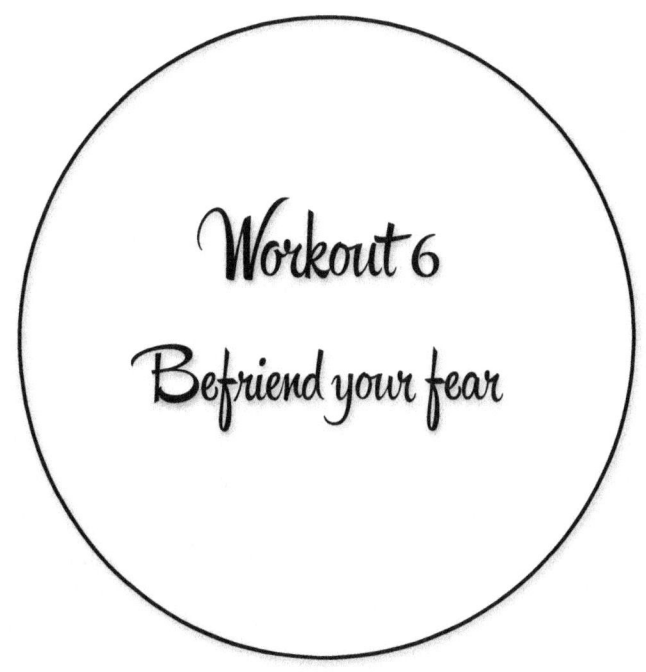

Workout 6

Befriend your fear

Many people make the mistake of thinking that confidence is the absence of fear. They try to avoid feeling fear, ignore it or pretend their fear is not there. But none of this helps them feel confident. Confidence comes when we learn to befriend our fear, not ignore it; when we let ourselves feel it and when we accept its presence. Confidence grows when we acknowledge the fear and still take action.

It is normal to feel fear. Fear is wired into us at a primal and physical level. When we lived in caves, fear was our inner warning system that helped us survive. It alerted us to sense physical danger and helped us protect ourselves.

The trouble is, not all fear is the same. We feel the same inner response for real physical danger as we do for perceived emotional risk — and mistakenly treat both in the same way.

If you are scared about presenting at a work meeting, even though you know all the data, this fear is different from physical fear where your life is in danger. It's emotional fear. It's based on a fear of emotional discomfort such as embarrassment, judgement or rejection, not on a fear for your life. It's based on perceived emotional danger, not real danger.

When we confuse the two we can mistakenly give a caveman response of fight or flight to situations that are emotional and in which these responses don't help. Neither response will help us feel confident.

Our flight reaction can make us hesitate when there is no need to hesitate. It makes us worry when we are prepared. It holds us back when we are ready. Our flight reaction makes us retreat unnecessarily and can leaves us questioning and doubting our own confidence.

Our fight reaction does the complete opposite, but is equally unhelpful. It makes us try to blast through fear as quickly as possible and not feel it. We try to soldier on. We use mental pump-ups and expressions such as 'Pull yourself together' and 'Just do it!' in an attempt to demand action of ourselves. But they are just bandaid solutions and do not give us confidence.

Soldiering on is a strategy for survival, but not very effective for building long-term confidence. You may get through that difficult meeting, but the next time you have to go to a difficult meeting you will find yourself back where you started, once again lacking confidence.

You don't want to just get through something; you want to become confident at it. You want to be able to repeat it, do it more than once and feel good when you do it.

Confidence does not come from trying to avoid feeling fear. It comes from acknowledging your fear and feeling it. Many people are scared to feel their fear because they mistakenly think that if they let themselves feel it, their fear will get worse. But that's not true. Feeling your fear does not make it worse. Feeling your fear helps you move through it and beyond it.

The next time you are about to do something for the first time and your fear rises up, put out a hand of compassion to yourself, not judgement. Remind yourself that whenever you start something new or end something familiar, it is normal to feel some level of fear. Change is a trigger for fear. When your fear arises simply reassure yourself with compassionate words such as, 'Of course I am scared, I've never done this before,' or 'Of course I'm scared, I'm stepping into something unknown.'

Fear is not your enemy. When it knocks at your door don't ignore it. Open the door, welcome it in and let it know that all emotions are welcome here. Open the door so you can learn why you are scared. Open the door to the details of your fear.

Don't say to yourself *I'm scared* and nothing more. You are not scared of everything. Take it deeper. Be more specific.

You can't take action against *I'm scared*. Saying you are scared just leaves you in a cloud of fog with nowhere to go. To take action, you need to clarify what exactly scares you. You need details about your fear.

Karen told me she was not confident driving to the city centre. She, like most of us, made the mistake of labelling her fear too broadly.

I said to her, 'Don't stop there. Dig deeper. Drill it down. Get clear on what specifically scares you.'

Is it the fast moving traffic?
Is it that you will get lost?
Is it that you can't read maps?
Is it being slow for other drivers?
Is it being on your own?
Is it that you are not a good driver?

When we force ourselves to articulate with precision what we are scared of, the fear moves from being something vague to something tangible; to something we can respond to and do something about.

You are not scared of everything. There are usually just one or two main factors that are holding you back. Once you realise you are not scared about every aspect of something, you can then start to see your way forward.

When Karen made herself be more specific she realised driving to the city centre was not the real fear. Getting lost was her real fear. That was something specific and tangible. Something she could see solutions to and take action to overcome. Something she felt confident to tackle.

The moment she knew her fear more specifically and in a tangible way, the ideas of how to boost her confidence became obvious. She could study maps of the city. She could ask someone to drive her there and show her around. She could give herself a day to drive to the city when she had time to get lost. She could even equip her car with a map, a mobile telephone, snacks, money and a full tank of petrol, so that she could let herself get lost without stress.

The actions that will build your confidence come from knowing and befriending your fear. Once you let yourself know your fear with more precision, the actions that lead to confidence suddenly become clear.

Ask yourself:

What response do you have when you feel fear?

How could you start to befriend your fear?

Fear is not your enemy. When it knocks at your door don't ignore it. Open the door and let it know it is welcome.

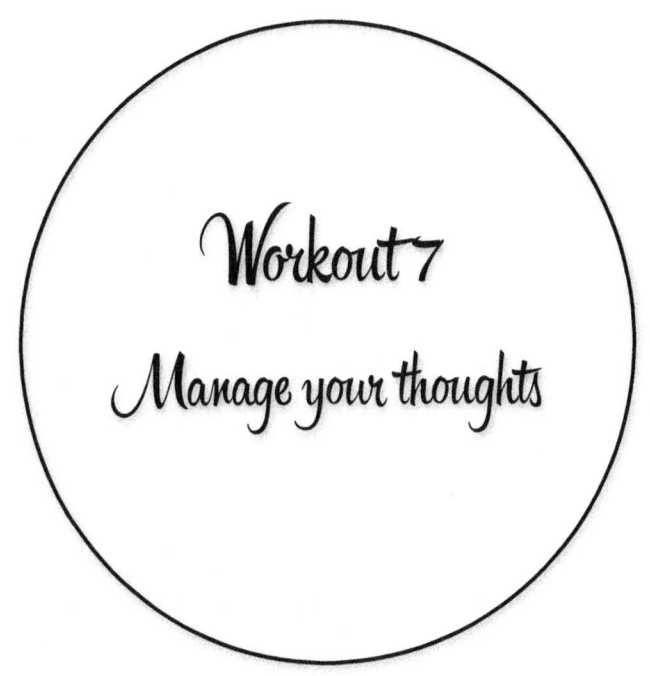

Workout 7

Manage your thoughts

Start listening to what you say to yourself. If you take a moment to properly listen to your own thinking you will be surprised to hear the many ways your thoughts undermine your confidence.

We tend to assume our thoughts are always true and accurate, but they aren't. Once you start listening to your thoughts you will quickly notice just how easily you can blow things out of proportion.

Our thoughts are often distortions and exaggerations of what is happening around us. They don't always reflect what is true and accurate. And sometimes our thoughts make things seem worse than they are in reality. We let our thoughts do this in many ways.

Sometimes we take something that is relatively neutral and turn it into something negative. We might trip over, but instead of simply thinking, 'I tripped over,' our thoughts can easily distort it and turn into something very different such as, 'I am clumsy,' 'I'm not coordinated,' or even, 'I can't do anything right.'

It is not the tripping over that robs us of our confidence; it is our thoughts about tripping over that do the damage.

Sometimes one small thing goes wrong, but we blow it out of proportion into something worse. One small hiccup can happen and we find ourselves reacting as if we are dealing with a major roadblock.

Sarah did this when she applied for a job in radio. When she received her first rejection letter, she instantly let her thoughts run out of control with exaggerated comments such as, 'Everything is going wrong', 'I always miss out,' and 'I'll never make it.'

Sometimes our minds exaggerate so much that that we are left thinking things that are simply not true. Sarah has received one rejection letter. That's all. *Everything* is not going wrong.

Whenever you hear yourself using words such as *everything, always* and *never,* be careful. These words are absolute and all-encompassing. Like a creeping mist, they can cover everything with negativity.

Our minds don't just exaggerate after events. We exaggerate beforehand, too. We can create doom and gloom scenarios and make ourselves believe these things are really going to happen.

That's what happened to David. I worked with him to help him feel more confident during work meetings. He kept losing his confidence before the meetings even began and it all came down to his thinking.

Before starting a meeting he would find himself thinking about all the things that could go wrong as if they certain and predetermined. He would let thoughts like 'What if I go blank in the middle of the meeting?' take hold and cripple his confidence before he even entered the room.

If you are like David and you hear yourself starting to think about all the things that might go wrong, you need to intercept your thoughts. But don't intercept by trying to stop your doom and gloom thoughts. Intercept and accentuate them. Exaggerate your worst-case scenario even more than you are already doing.

This may sound strange, but you want to break the pattern of exaggeration and the best way to do this is to consciously exaggerate.

If you hear yourself blowing things out of proportion and thinking of all the things that might go wrong, don't let your mind half do it. Make yourself play out your full nightmare. Unravel your fear.

When your mind starts thinking, 'What if I go blank in the middle of the meeting?' don't stop the story there. Make yourself articulate your nightmare scenario. Let your mind play it out fully.

'When I go blank, I will look stupid, then everyone will stare at me, then I will go red, then my boss will tell me I no longer have a job, then I will burst out crying in front of everyone, then I will have no money, then I will lose my house, then I will be homeless …'

Keep going until your nightmare scenario seems ridiculous. At a certain point you realise going blank will not make you homeless. At a certain point you will know this is just your thoughts and the story in your head that is scaring you, not what will happen.

Exaggerating breaks the spell our thinking has over us. It makes us conscious of what our mind is doing subconsciously. It frees us to choose positive and more confident ways of thinking.

Most of us try to be positive too quickly. We need to first completely unravel the worst-case story before we rewrite a positive one. No amount of positive thinking on the surface will boost your confidence if underneath that your doom and gloom thoughts continue.

Thank goodness the way we think is just a habit and we can change it easily. It all starts with how we see our mind and what we expect of our mind.

To change your thoughts you need to stop assuming your mind is doing its best. It's not! Your mind is often just repeating learnt patterns of thinking. It's not trying to think the best way it can. Most of the time your mind is just on automatic.

If your automatic programming is positive and builds your confidence, then being on automatic is fine. But if your programming is not supportive of what you want to do, switch into manual mode.

Most of us give our minds too much free range. We let our own thoughts erode our confidence, letting them go where they like, when they like. We let worry-filled thoughts bombard us without restraint. We forget that our mind makes a wonderful slave, but a terrible master.

A great way to stop confidence-crushing thoughts bombarding every moment of your day is to set up an appointment time to do all your worrying. When you mind starts thinking of all the things that might go wrong and screams out 'what if I go blank?' simply say back to yourself, 'Let's worry about that at five o'clock tonight, not now.'

Let the fearful part of you know it will be heard, but it cannot just butt in. Let your doom and gloom voice rise up and have an outlet, but at a time that suits you. At a time that does not erode your confidence.

Scheduling an appointment for worry not only controls your doom and gloom voice, it quietens it too. Your doom and gloom voice does not know how to talk in restrained ways and at set times. It is used to interrupting, barging in and taking over. Invariably at five o'clock it won't have much to say.

Ask yourself:

When have you blown things out of proportion and undermined your confidence?

What could you do differently next time your doom and gloom voice starts to talk?

When you start thinking of all the things that might go wrong, don't let your mind half do it. Play out your full nightmare.

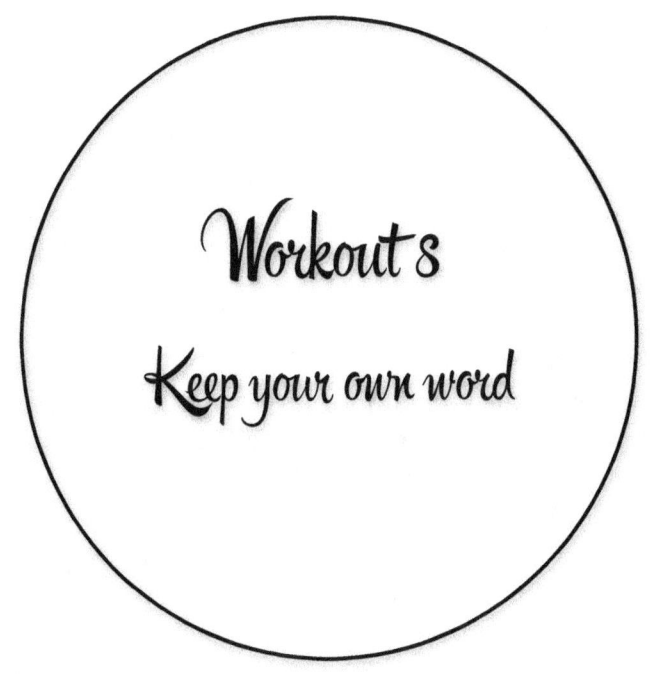

Workout 8

Keep your own word

Sometimes in our eagerness to achieve a goal we set unrealistic plans about how we are going to get there. We set out with big intentions and bold plans based on what we would like to do without first assessing how realistic the plan is given our other commitments, given the structure of our lives and given that the pursuit may be a completely new habit that takes time to build into those factors.

We decide we want to get fit and boldly say things like 'I am going to walk for two hours every day this week,' only to find we don't do it.

That is exactly what Tanya did. She didn't fully consider the realities of her life when setting her goal to start exercising. She told everyone she was going to start going to the gym five days a week, but ended up only going once a week.

Not doing what you say may seem inconsequential, but it isn't. It will silently erode your confidence. Every time you say you will do something and then don't, you erode your self-trust; you give up a little on yourself, you stop trusting your own word and you stop feeling like you can count on yourself.

After a few weeks Tanya started to lose confidence that she would ever achieve her goal of losing weight. And as she lost confidence in herself and her plans, she started going to the gym less and less until eventually she gave up.

It is great to have big intentions, but only if you follow through with action. Set big plans and big goals, but only say you will do something if you really will do it. If you don't, over time you risk damaging the most important relationship you have: the one of self-trust.

To feel confident you need to keep your word with yourself. You need to set plans that you can do and commit to actions that you will achieve.

Once you start keeping your word with yourself you'll be surprised at how quickly you start to feel confident in what you are doing. Being more realistic won't slow you down. In the end it will get you there more quickly. That's because you will stay confident and actually do what you commit to.

Tanya decided to revise her whole approach to exercise. She put 'keeping her word' central to her plan knowing that maintaining her confidence in herself and in her ability to achieve her goal was central to achieving it.

She set realistic targets and set an amount that she was sure she could do. She set shorter session times and gave herself two days off each week. She exercised in the mornings and stopped expecting herself to exercise after work when she was tired.

By designing a plan that fit her rhythms and the realities of her life, she finally started to keep her word and start exercising. Not only did she rebuild her confidence, it wasn't long before she was also achieving her goal of becoming fitter and losing weight.

Think about one of your goals and some actions that would be realistic for you. Don't ignore the realities of your life and the things that make achieving your goals harder. Work with them. Consider them. Put realism right into the core of your action plan and so that you plan a way to take action considering your life, as it is.

Separate what you would love to do versus what you can and will realistically do. You may want to walk for two hours every day this week, but you also need to ask yourself whether it is practically possible. If you work, your husband is away and you have children, then it may not be realistic to walk that far this week.

Make doing what you say more important than trying to do anything big. Setting big goals is great if you are certain you will do big actions too. But if in doubt, don't put your self-trust and confidence at risk. When it comes to confidence it is better to start small and be sure you do it than to project too big and end up doing nothing.

Start with what you absolutely know you can do and will do. If you want to walk for two hours every day, then start by committing to walking for twenty minutes or an amount you are certain you can do. If you manage to walk for more, then that's great, but at least if you don't walk more you have kept your word and therefore your confidence as well.

Always make keeping your word your first priority. Once you have built your confidence, in both your commitment and in what you are doing, then you can expand the quantity you promise yourself to do.

Your promises to yourself do impact your confidence. Therefore, if you say you will do something, make sure you fully intend to do it. Don't let it be something that gets done if there is time at the end of your day. Schedule it in your diary. Use ink, not pencil. Treat it like it matters by making it less moveable.

Ask yourself:

When have you not kept your word to yourself?

What would be realistic for you to commit to?

Keep your own word with yourself. It feeds your confidence when you know you can count on yourself.

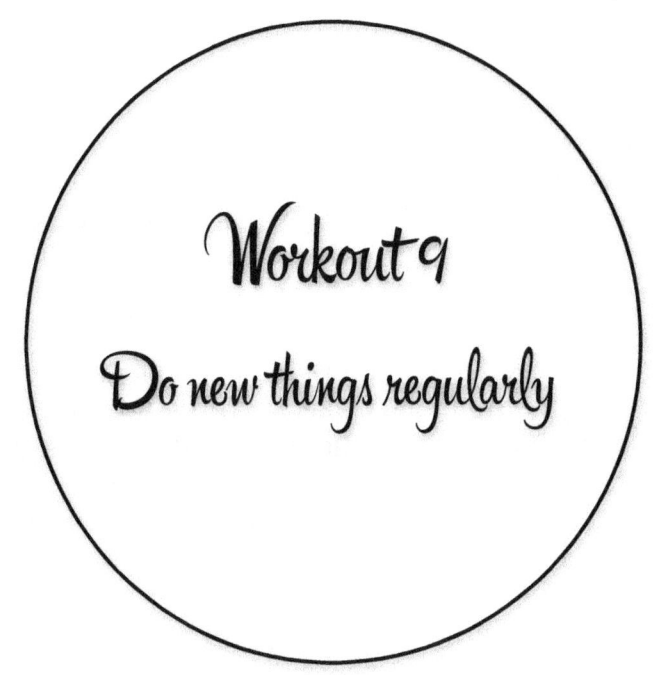

Workout 9

Do new things regularly

When I was eight years old I remember my teacher telling us he was leaving the school. I was devastated. I couldn't imagine another teacher being as good as him. I cried my heart out. I was scared about who would replace him, but then to my surprise the next teacher was also fantastic.

This happens to us all the time. We mistakenly think what we have is as good as it gets. We even have an expression for it, 'Better the devil you know than the one you don't!'

Thinking this way restricts us enormously. Sticking with the devil you know is not always better. It makes us stick with the known, even when the known is bad. It makes us not even evaluate other options and not even try other things.

It can make us overstay too. 'Better the devil you know' thinking makes us overstay in jobs, relationships and situations that often no longer match where we want to be. It makes us restrict our lives to the tried and tested and confine ourselves to what is familiar and known.

The pull towards familiarity is strong in most of us. People through all time and cultures have gravitated to what is known. In ancient cultures it was a survival mechanism.

The unknown meant possible danger and the known meant safety. Yet in today's modern world sticking to only what is familiar is often misplaced and unnecessarily limiting. It makes us restrict our lives, only doing the things that we feel confident and familiar doing. We do the same things over and over, never daring to venture outside these known boundaries.

Sticking to what is familiar can give us the illusion of confidence, but that's because we only do what we are already confident doing!

If you are like most people, you want to be able to do new things. You want a fulfilling life and there are all sorts of things you would love to try, experiences you would like to have and places you would like to go. But to do these things you have to step beyond what is familiar and develop your confidence with newness.

To be confident with new things, you need to make *doing new things* become familiar and a part of your everyday life. You don't have to leap out and do something new that is big and scary to do. That's the beauty of developing confidence; it can be done in small and simple ways to prepare us for the big things.

Janette came to see me because she wanted to travel to Finland to attend a conference, but she had never been overseas before and the idea of going to a new country by herself scared her. For years she had kept familiarity at the centre of her life.

Going to the conference was a big leap; too big for someone who did not have confidence in doing anything new. First she had to become comfortable with new things in easy ways and everyday ways. If she was to do this trip with confidence, she needed to start doing lots of small new things before doing something big. She had to make newness itself became familiar.

She set herself the challenge of doing something new every day. After two weeks she came to see me with a long list of new little things she had done. She had travelled to work in different ways. She had tried out new restaurants and ordered dishes she had never eaten before. She had her hair cut by a different hairdresser. She even started saying hello to people in her street that previously she had just walked past.

Her confidence soared. Suddenly, the unfamiliar became easy and manageable. The more new little things she did, the more confident she started to feel about doing her trip to Finland. Week by week she increasingly began to trust that her world wouldn't fall apart just because she was doing something new.

Try this in your life. Find ways to sprinkle newness through your life.

Read a book you would not normally read.
Listen to different types of music from normal.
Voice an opinion you wouldn't normally give.
Say hello to someone you don't know.
Cook something you wouldn't normally cook.

Drive home a different route.
Clean your teeth with the opposite hand.
Sleep in the spare bed instead of your own.
Wear an outfit you haven't worn for ages.
Catch a train instead of the bus.

You may add newness into your life by taking up a new activity, but often the easiest way to sprinkle newness through your life is to do an existing activity a different way. Work out what habit might be fun to change temporarily. You want to make doing new things interesting and positive.

Ask yourself:

How comfortable are you doing new things?

What new things could you start doing in your life?

To feel confident to do big new things, it helps to do little new things in your everyday life.

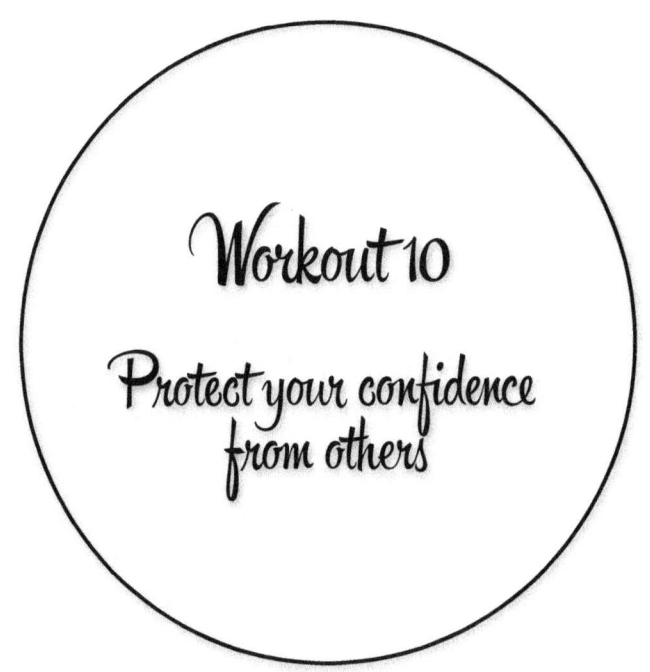

Workout 10

Protect your confidence from others

Most of us were brought up with the saying, 'Sticks and stones will break your bones, but words will never hurt you.' However, when it comes to confidence this expression is not entirely true — words can hurt us. They hurt our confidence.

Other people's comments and remarks can have a big influence on our confidence if we let them. And sometimes we put our confidence at risk by not managing our relationships with negative people very well.

You won't ever be able to stop all the negative comments that come your way from others, but you can influence how you respond to them; how you protect yourself, how you manage the interaction and how much time you spend with negative people. You can reduce how much you expose yourself to people who crush your confidence and you can learn to reduce their influence over how you feel and not let their negative comments stick.

Our confidence is special and valuable and needs to be cared for. Sometimes it needs protection. Unfortunately however, we don't always guard our confidence well enough. We put up with toxic comments from others, not realising just how easily words can pierce our confidence and how impacting even just a few remarks can be.

When the ties run deep we often put up with their confidence-crushing comments too readily. These comments can come from family or friends whom we have known for years. Sometimes these people are woven into the fabric of our lives — parents, brothers, sisters, aunties, uncles, bosses and colleagues. They are people we see regularly and have to interact with in our daily life.

If you are like most people there will be someone in your life who, if you let them, could undermine your confidence. Their statements to you may be blatant put-downs, although often they are subtler. They can be less of a blow, yet more ongoing, with continual snide remarks or discouraging comments.

Sometimes we don't realise the impact others have on our confidence until the damage is done or until someone's cutting remark has already cut.

Sometimes we try to brush their comment aside as if it did not matter. Occasionally we even justify their ways saying, 'That's just how they are.' But despite our excuses for their behaviour their comments still impact us.

Sally had a circle of friends who were constantly putting her down. It took her a while to realise what was happening. After years of spending time with them, their put-downs and negativity had become commonplace; so familiar that she hardly noticed. But her self esteem noticed. When she spent time with them she felt disempowered and less confident about everything she did.

Sometimes we notice our confidence slip immediately in someone's presence. There is a stabbing impact from their comments that affects how we feel. Other times we don't notice until afterwards, when we are alone again and then realise we are filled with doubt and less sure about what we were doing earlier that day.

You'll know if others are having a toxic effect on your confidence by how you feel after spending time with them. If every time you spend time with them you feel depleted or emotionally drained, it's a sign to change the impact they have on you.

Think about the people in your life. Who pulls you down? Who discourages you? Who depletes your confidence?

Become mindful of the different impact people in your life have on you. If there are people who are eroding your confidence, you need to start to protect it. You need to value how you feel and take steps to change the influence they have on how you feel.

Guarding your confidence from others does not mean dropping the negative people completely from your life. However, stopping contact may be what you initially need to do while you rebuild your confidence. Mostly though, you don't have to drop people. You just have to drop the influence they have over you.

You cannot always control the things people say to you, but you can control your response. You can choose what you take on, what you let stick. You can choose how much time you will spend with them and how much interaction you have. You can choose to stop allowing their put-downs as an acceptable way to speak to you.

Nobody can put us down unless we allow them to. Sometimes we inadvertently allow others to erode our confidence through what we do and what we don't do. If we listen, week in and week out, to someone putting us down, and say nothing and do nothing, then we are allowing them to erode our confidence. Our silence condones it. Our presence accepts it.

If you keep listening to put-downs from someone, unless you are locked in a prison cell together, then chances are you are allowing it. As Eleanor Roosevelt so famously said, 'No one can make you feel inferior without your consent.'

Your confidence is precious. It is hard won and easily lost. Value it. Protect it. Don't keep putting yourself in situations that allow others to slay it.

To do the things you want to be confident doing, you need people who build you up rather than tear you down. Think about whom you surround yourself with and start choosing to spend more time with people who nurture and nourish your confidence. If you truly want to feel confident you don't want to just manage the negative people in your life, you want to fill your life with positive people.

Ask yourself:

Who in your life has a negative impact on your confidence?

How do you allow them to impact your confidence?

You cannot always control the things people say to you, but you can control your response.

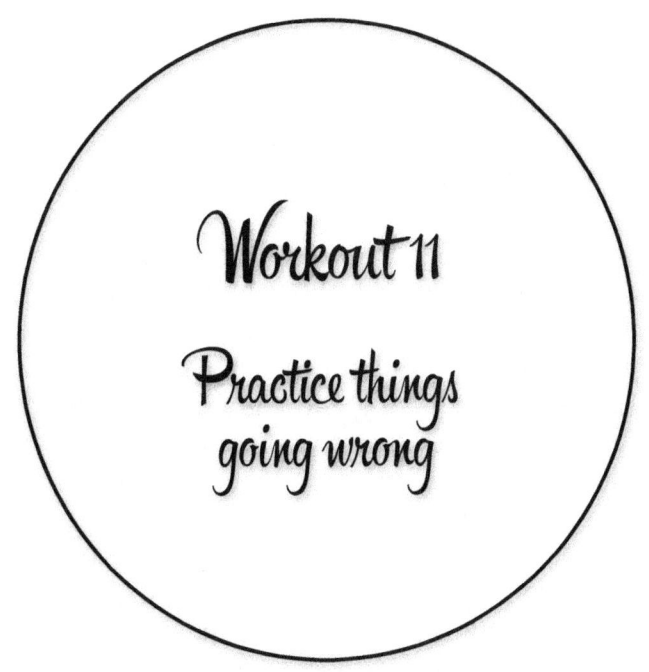

Workout 11

Practice things going wrong

Confidence does not come from knowing you can do something with perfect conditions around you. It comes from knowing you can cope and respond when you have all the wrong conditions.

We feel confident when we know we are resourceful and can adapt when things go wrong. We feel it when we know we are capable of adjusting what we are doing if things around us change.

However, most of us don't practice in ways that develop our resourcefulness and confidence. We practise our pursuits in perfect environments with perfect conditions, and inadvertently train ourselves to only feel confident when everything around us is perfect.

This happened to me when I first learnt to cook as a teenager. I diligently followed exactly what was written in recipe books. Over time I learnt to cook reasonably well, but my skills were always conditional on having the right ingredients and having available the equipment stated in the recipes. I had learnt to cook competently, but not confidently.

This became evident one evening when I was halfway through preparing a dish and I realised I was missing carrots. I had no idea what to use as a substitute ingredient. And instead of adapting, I abandoned making that dish.

I was missing more than an ingredient; I was missing the confidence to improvise and adjust what I was doing. I didn't know how to adapt the recipe, as I had no practice in adapting.

If the only time you do your pursuit is when you have perfect conditions, your confidence will not be fully developed. It will be conditional and it won't take much for it to disappear — as soon as one element disappears so will your confidence.

To develop your adaptability, you need to give yourself opportunities to be adaptable. You need to weave it into how you practise your skills.

You need practice in a non-perfect environment, not just a perfect environment. You need to practise things going wrong, not just going right. You need to practise with items not working, missing and elements deteriorating around you.

Think about how you do your practice sessions. How could you fill your practice sessions with non-perfect conditions? What elements could you let go wrong? How can you strengthen your adaptability and your confidence?

Fill your practice sessions with non-perfect conditions. Set up the problem scenarios and simulate things going wrong.

This is what airline pilots do. In the simulators they practice flying with everything going wrong, not right. This broadens their skills and gives them the confidence to respond and cope if something ever happens in the middle of a real flight.

If you are learning to paddle a kayak, don't just practise staying in the kayak; practise falling out. Practise recovering, practise tipping the boat near the shore in smooth water, in choppy water and even with your eyes closed.

Practise what you fear most. Allow all the things you hope will never happen to happen. If you are worried about your projector failing in the middle of your presentation, then practise having it fail in the middle of a rehearsal.

Place your confidence in your adaptability, not in the power supply. Then if there are power problems in the middle of your real presentation and your projector stops working, you will have the confidence to keep going. It's our adaptability, not our control that makes us feel most confident.

Practice in diverse ways. Every time you do your pursuit, do one thing differently.

Try new combinations, new ingredients and new sequences. Practise in different settings and under different conditions. Do it faster, slower or even backwards. Each time change one element.

You want your confidence to be anchored in your resourcefulness and adaptability, not in the conditions around you. After all, you don't want your confidence to evaporate just because you are missing some carrots.

Ask yourself:

How can you practise things going wrong and build your resourcefulness?

How can you practise in new and different ways?

Practise what
you fear most.
Allow the things
you hope will
never happen to
happen.

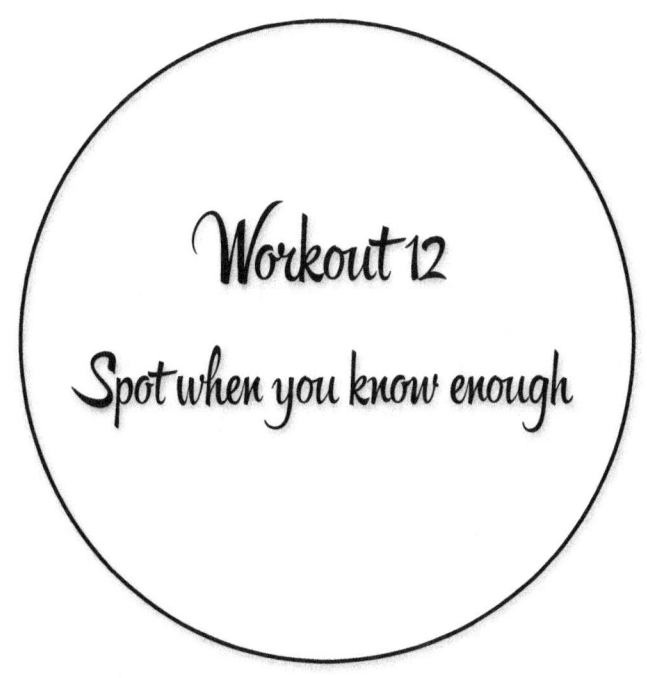

Workout 12

Spot when you know enough

Sometimes we won't take action until we are literally spilling over with knowledge. We mistakenly think we have to know *everything* to be ready and then set ourselves up to never feel confident enough to take that next step.

If knowing everything becomes your basis for feeling confident and your launching ground for action, you may never feel ready to start. It's impossible to feel ready; that's because you can never know *everything*.

Knowledge is infinite. Trying to know everything is like climbing into a bottomless pit; the more you know, the more you discover there is to know. It has no end.

Don't get me wrong, knowledge is important. You need to know *something* about what you are doing. You need to know quite a bit to take action. And sometimes, depending on the pursuit, you will need to know a massive amount.

The question you must ask yourself is *'How much is enough?'*

Charlie had developed quite a reputation for his successful alternate medical treatments. During one of his coaching sessions he told he had been invited to present at an international conference to talk about his treatments. 'It is a dream come true,' he admitted, 'but I'm not confident enough to do it. I still don't know everything there is to know.'

Charlie's relationship with his own knowledge was holding him back. Charlie was knowledgeable and had a lot to offer the audience, but his relationship with his knowledge was blocking him from his own confidence. He had linked his confidence to the unachieveable goal of 'having to know everything'.

We need to manage our relationship with our own knowledge carefully. Knowing things *does* boost our confidence, but not as much as we often think. It only boosts it in the early stages.

When we are going from no knowledge to some knowledge, that's when knowing more boosts our confidence the most. Every little bit we learn helps us feel more confident about what we are doing and what is possible to do. But the impact more knowledge has on our confidence does not go up forever. Soon the confidence benefits start to plateau and even subside.

Once you know a lot, that's when you most need to remind yourself that you will never know everything. That's what Charlie had to do. He had to realise that he would never get a *now I know it all moment,* and that by thinking there was one, he was sabotaging his confidence.

Thinking there is a *now I know it all moment* stops us in many ways. It stops us noticing what we do know. It stops us noticing how we are already ready for action. Above all else, it keeps us in an endless cycle of preparation.

Thinking there is a *now I know it all moment* makes us hesitate when in reality we may be ready to take our next step. It makes us over prepare. It makes us more likely to gather obsessively.

Research obsessively. Practice obsessively. But our preparation has no end and our confidence wavers in its wake.

Your dream pursuit may need you to gather lots of knowledge and expertise. You may need to do years of study and research. But the secret to confident action is to not place your confidence in knowing *everything*. The secret is to know when you know enough.

Change the question you ask yourself. You will never feel confident if you ask yourself if you know everything. Instead ask yourself whether you know enough.

Do you know enough to start?
Do you now enough to take action?
Do you know enough to give it a go?

Some pursuits you do may have an in-built *now you know enough* point set by others. A university course often has this; after five years of study and 45 exams passed you are deemed ready. Ready to take action. Ready to take the next step. Ready to be confident. This can make it easier to take action even when you are not yet confident.

But what about the pursuits that have no measurable or definable *now you know enough* point deemed by an institute, by a job title or by someone else? You may have to be the person who has to decide when you are at your *now I know enough to start* point.

Let yourself delight in knowing and learning more, because wanting to know more is empowering and motivates us forward. However, trying to know everything does the opposite. It makes us feel inadequate, hesitant and makes us hold back. It erodes our confidence.

Ask yourself:

Have you been waiting to know everything about your pursuit before taking action?

Do you know enough to start?

Don't ask yourself
if you know
everything. Instead
ask yourself if you
know enough.

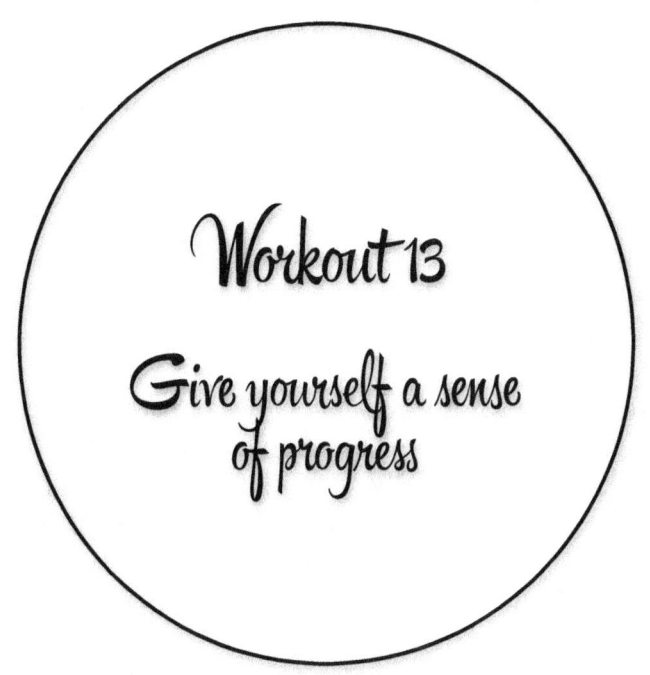

Workout 13

Give yourself a sense of progress

If you chip away at something slowly and feel like you are getting nowhere, it's not only disheartening; it is hard to keep feeling confident. Confidence is fed when we feel like we are making progress.

Having a sense of progress nourishes our confidence. In turn, this motivates us to keep going. It helps us to keep trying despite our mistakes and keep persisting even when the learning curve is steep.

Lisa had been learning to dance for a few months when I met her. She had always wanted to learn and had never had the opportunity as a child. She told me, 'I was confident when I started, but now it's quickly fading.'

Her voice filled with frustration as she blurted out, 'I'm thinking of giving up. I'm not making any progress at all. I don't think I will ever be able to dance well.'

'You've forgotten how far you have come,' I said. 'When you started you didn't dance at all. Now look how beautifully you move. Look at all the dance steps you now know. You are losing your confidence simply because you have no sense of your own progress.'

Like many of our pursuits, her pursuit has no obvious progress points. There are no 'now you can dance' achievement points and marker points for comparison. Her improvement is subtle, continual and so incremental that it is hard to spot from one moment to the next.

When we do a pursuit regularly we often adjust to our improvements without noticing them. Each day we become slightly better, but it is so incremental that it is hard to see. We have no gaps in time to notice our progress. We are too close and our perspective is too frequent.

Progress can be subtle. The improvements we make from one day to the next can be hard to spot. Often we are indeed making progress, but we just can't see the gains we've made.

Some pursuits, like learning a foreign language, don't have black and white achievement points. You learn a few more words. You use these words in more situations. You learn to string different words together. The progress is happening but it is grey and hard to measure.

If your pursuit has no obvious progress points, find a way to make your progress more definable and noticeable. Don't leave the sense of progress to chance. Build it in. Make it obvious.

Make your progress obvious by noticing what you get right. You will get some things wrong and some things right. What you choose to notice and focus on is what will influence your confidence to keep going.

When Jack became interested in gardening, he built a vegetable garden in his back yard. As a beginner at growing vegetables he planted an assortment of vegetables. At the end of summer he told me half the plants had died and the other half had grown well and produced vegetables.

He could have told me what didn't work and say, 'I'm not good at gardening because half my plants died,' but he didn't. He fed his confidence by noticing what worked and told me, 'I'm progressing well. Half my crop produced vegetables.'

Learn to notice the little things you do well and where you are improving, even if they seem insignificant and even if the overall outcome is not good.

If you are working toward becoming an artist, find one corner of your drawing that you like. If you are working toward becoming a freelance journalist, find one paragraph of your article that was written well. If you are trying to become a better runner, notice one part of your training workout that you did with perfect focus. No matter how small, let these little markers be the foundation upon which you build a sense of progress and your confidence.

Each week ask yourself what you can now do that you couldn't do last week. Ask yourself questions that make you reflect.

What am I getting right?
What did I do well?
What did I do that I want to keep doing?

Children are masters at this. When my son was learning to count he loved reading mailbox numbers. The first time he read them, he only got a few right, but he came home telling everyone he got three numbers right. His focus was exclusively on what he got right.

Each day he got a few more right and each day he focused only on what he got right. By completely ignoring his errors he was filled with a huge sense of progress and his confidence soared. And before long he was getting them all right.

A great way to give yourself a sense of progress is to capture what your skills are when you start. This will give you a comparison point for later; something you can refer back to as indisputable proof that you are indeed making progress.

Try this. Whatever your pursuit is, capture where you are at now before it changes too much. Document and highlight where your skills are now before you get too much traction and before it changes. Capture your lack of skill, your lack of mastery or even your lack of confidence.

Capture these aspects in a format that will give you evidence later. If you are learning to windsurf, you could ask someone to video your first attempts. If you are learning to draw, you could keep your first charcoal drawings. If you are learning the piano, you could write out a 'this is what I can do now' statement or record yourself playing.

Make sure you capture as much detail as possible. If you are writing a description of your current skills, be specific. Write down, 'I can play one tune on the piano; it has four notes and I can only use one hand.'

Then later when you think you are not making progress get out the video, get out the drawings or read the comments you wrote. Immerse yourself in those beginner moments and show yourself that you now stand in a different place.

Ask yourself:

How can you create a sense of progress?

What will best capture your progress?

No matter how small, notice your progress and let it be the foundation upon which you build your confidence.

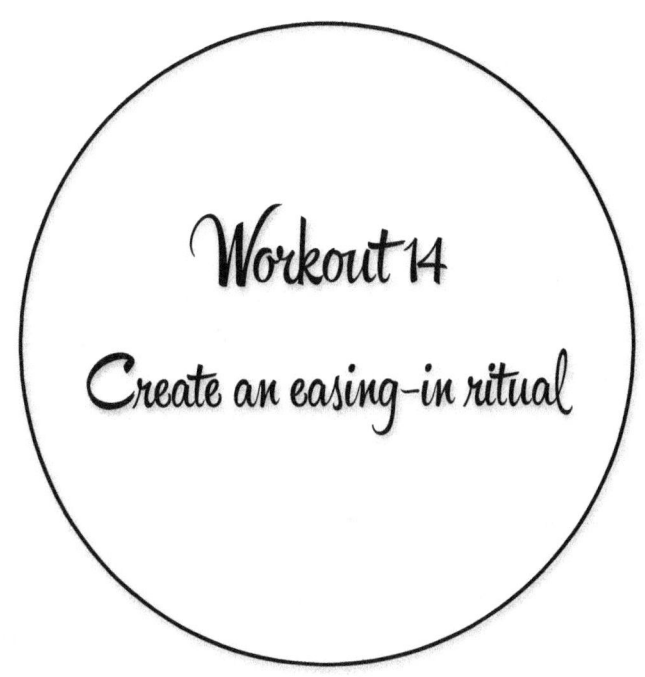

Workout 14

Create an easing-in ritual

Whenever we have a large break from a pursuit our confidence seems to take a dive. We often struggle to return to the flow that we ended with a few months earlier.

My friend Carol is a painter. When she is in the flow of painting every day she finds she can naturally reconnect to her confidence each morning. She easily picks up where she left off the day before. But when she takes a break of even just a few weeks this all changes. Sometimes when she returns to her work, she feels like her confidence has completely disappeared.

This happens when we have a large break from anything. The larger the break, the more likely we will feel this loss of confidence.

It may feel like your confidence has disappeared, but it hasn't. It is your connection to your confidence that has gone, not your confidence itself. When you look closer nothing has happened to dismantle it. Just time.

The easiest way to keep our confidence alive is to do our pursuits in a regular rhythm, without large breaks in time. Breaks in time disconnect us from our flow and from our self-belief. However for most of us, it is not possible to do our pursuits in continuation. Breaks are inevitable.

Breaks are not such a problem however, if you don't expect to be able to pick up where you left off. If you attempt to go straight to action, without connecting to your confidence, it often makes you think your skills, creativity and talent have disappeared too, when none of these actually have. And you may risk thinking that you are no longer good at your art form, when in reality you just do not know how to reconnect to it.

Make reconnection to your confidence the first thing you do on return. Create an easing-in ritual where the focus is to reconnect you to your pursuit. It does not have to be complicated at all, just something that eases you back into action without any pressure or judgement.

Musicians naturally do this when they do their scales. You may think they are just physically warming up, but scales do much more. They help musicians establish their flow before they tackle more complex music.

Athletes don't start their races cold, either. Before a race, you'll see most athletes do a short sequence of stretches and movement. It is always the same sequence. Their starting rituals help them make the transition smoothly from no action to intense performance.

I have an easing-in ritual I do when I have not written for a while. It helps me reconnect to the writer in me. I have an inspirational song that I play and then I spend a few minutes reading previous writing out loud. When I pick up my pen I remove all pressure and let myself ease back in by writing a page of scribble and ideas.

Your easing-in ritual does not have to be long and complicated. In fact, sometimes the shorter it is the quicker it connects you to your confidence.

There are a thousand different ways to reconnect to your confidence. It's up to you what you choose, but there are some important elements that will help you reconnect to your confidence faster.

Make your ritual repetitive. Do the same ritual every time you want to reconnect. The repetitive nature of doing the same thing increases the association between doing that ritual and feeling confident. Like a light switch being turned on, your body and mind will associate this ritual with confidence.

Remove all pressure. When you first start your activity, start in a way that allows you to remove all worry about the quality of your work and what you are doing. Make your sole focus reconnection to your confidence, not performance.

Don't give your judging self any opportunity to speak up. Critiquing and editing can come later. When starting, remove all judgement, as it will stop you accessing your confidence.

Don't expect high performance immediately. When you sit down to paint after a one-month break, don't expect to be able to just dive back into creating a perfect painting. Ease yourself back in. Make ease your priority. Once you are in your flow, then you can increase the complexity.

Choose a ritual that matches your personality. Each of us is different so our ritual needs to match who we are. If you like music, include uplifting songs. If you find visual images uplifting, flick through photos of you doing your pursuit before starting.

Make your ritual similar to your pursuit. If you are trying to reconnect to running, reading will probably not help you. There is not enough common ground. But if you are sitting down to write, reading is in a similar realm.

There should be a logical link between how you start and the pursuit you are doing. You need to ease-in in a way that is similar enough to allow you to flow straight into your pursuit. The ritual acts as a bridge.

Ask yourself:

What starting ritual would help you connect to your confidence?

What elements should you include because they match both your personality and your pursuit?

It may feel like your confidence has disappeared, but it hasn't. It is your connection to your confidence that has gone, not your confidence itself.

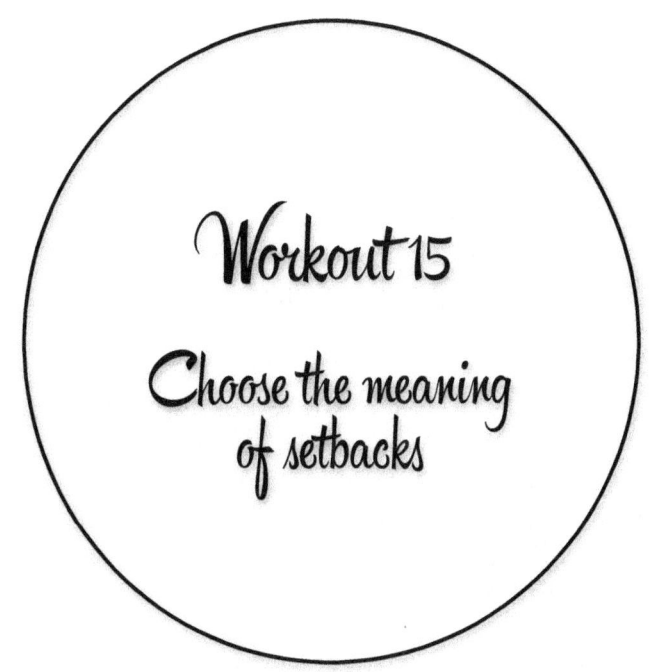

Workout 15

Choose the meaning of setbacks

There is a magical window of opportunity that exists immediately after any setback we may have. Our reaction to what could be a setback has not yet been locked into memory and therefore our mind is still pliable. We remain open to new and varied meanings.

What you say to yourself in that moment straight after a setback is vital, because what you say impacts how confident you will feel. It will make you either want to give up or help you to bounce back.

Most of us let ourselves down in that moment. We don't seize the opportunity to steer our thinking and influence our own confidence. Instead we invariably let our minds spiral out of control, creating all sorts of negative meanings about what has just happened.

It's not the event that determines if we will bounce back or not, it's the meaning we choose to give to the event that determines it. That's because meaning is not fixed in stone. It is something we give to things. If we want to keep our confidence intact we can choose positive and helpful meanings.

My daughter is a keen horse rider. One day when she was still little and hadn't been riding for long, her horse bucked her off in the middle of a lesson. She was unhurt, but as she lay there on the ground I knew she was at the crossroads of two distinctly different responses: either bounce back or give up.

Being a beginner, it would have been easy for her to personalise the fall and say to herself, 'I'm a terrible rider. I'm not good enough. I'll never learn.' But before she had time to create any negative meanings from the situation, her instructor yelled out, 'Now you are closer to being a real rider. They always say you have to fall off seven times before you can call yourself a real rider.'

A smile swept across my daughter's face and she stood up, ready to ride again.

When you next have a setback, step into this window of opportunity and choose a positive meaning. Give yourself a chance to bounce back by saying things to yourself that make it easier to pick yourself back up.

It does not matter if comments like *you have to fall off your horse seven times to be a real rider* are true or not. What matters is whether they are helpful or not.

If you want to feel confident, it's up to you to choose meanings that help this happen. You can choose the meaning you give to any setback, obstacle or mistake. And what you choose determines how you will feel.

We can learn a lot from Thomas Edison and the meanings he made on his journey to inventing the light bulb. Even though he made many failed attempts to invent the light bulb, he never saw his attempts as failures.

He saw every invention that didn't work as an opportunity for further insight. He saw every wrong discovery as an opportunity to learn what wouldn't work. As a consequence his confidence stayed solid and strong.

The secret to bouncing back lies in choosing to find a positive meaning out of any attempt, mistake or setback you have. When you were little you did this all the time.

When you were learning to talk you made many mistakes and failed to speak correctly many times. You said things the wrong way. You pronounced words incorrectly. Sometimes nobody understood you at all. But you were not deterred.

You kept your confidence intact because you had not yet learnt to see failure as anything other than feedback. You had no negative associations and had not yet seen mistakes as a reason to give up

Intuitively you used your mistakes as guideposts that highlighted what not to do. Each wrong pronunciation was simply feedback to help you learn how to pronounce that word better the next time.

Seize the window of opportunity that exists to make positive meaning out of everything that happens. Help yourself bounce back by saying things that nurture your confidence instead of destroying it.

The next time you have a setback, stop and take notice of what you are saying to yourself.

If you can feel yourself thinking about giving up, intercept your thoughts and ask yourself:

What else could this mean?
What meaning will best serve me right now?
What meaning will help me to stay confident?

Nothing has meaning of its own. You get to choose the meaning of everything that happens to you. Give yourself a chance to feel confident and choose a meaning that feeds your confidence.

Ask yourself:

When have you had a setback and let it erode your confidence?

What more helpful meaning could you have chosen?

Michelle Landy

Nothing has
meaning of its
own. You get
to choose the
meaning of
everything that
happens to you.

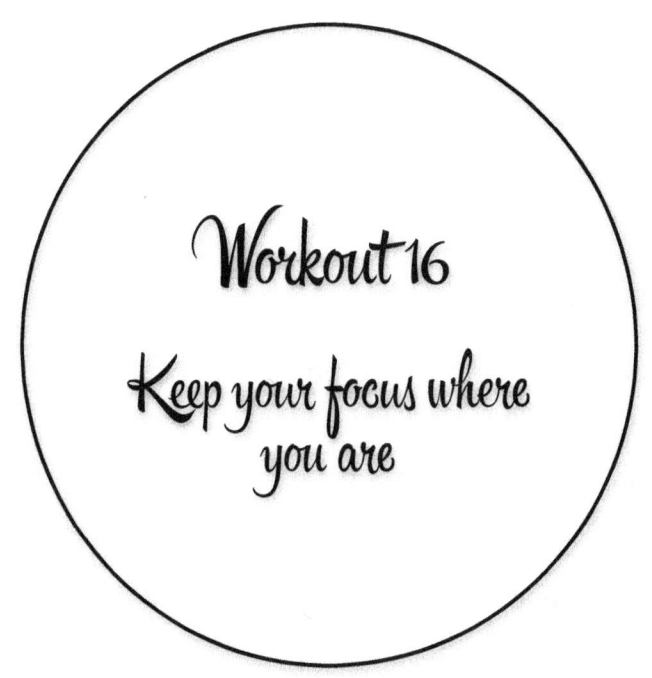

Workout 16

Keep your focus where you are

Keep your eye on the goal. That's what most of us have been taught to do. However, when it comes to keeping our confidence alive, keeping our eye on the goal can be the worst place to put our attention.

If your pursuit is big and hard to achieve, keeping your eye on the goal can overwhelm you and make it hard for you to feel confident. If you keep your eye only on the goal you highlight the gap between where you are now and where you want to be. It accentuates how much there is to do and how hard it will be. None of which helps you feel confident.

There is no doubt you need to know your goal and need to know where you are heading. After all, your goal is your magnet that helps you move forward. However, to sustain your confidence as you progress, it is better to make your goal a reference point, not your everyday focus point.

Your confidence is kept stronger when you create closer destination points, halfway markers and mini arrival points along the way. Confidence is a present time feeling so the closer your focus is to what you are doing right now, the more it will help you feel confident.

If you want to write a book of poems, don't overwhelm yourself by focusing on how you will write one hundred poems. Focus on writing just the poem you want to write today. If you want to lose weight, instead of focusing on what you will have to eat for the next six months, just focus on what you will eat today.

The steps ahead of you do matter and yes, it is wise to prepare for them. Plan, organise and get yourself ready for those steps in the future, but then bring your focus back to where you are now; to what you are doing right now and what you can respond to right now, because confidence lies in present time.

If you are climbing a mountain you need to prepare the right gear for the journey, know the crevices and terrain and prepare for all the steps of the journey. However, when you actually start climbing your focus needs to shift. You need to put your attention on what you are doing each moment along the way. To stay confident you need to keep your attention on the crevice in front of you right now and not be worrying about the ones ahead of you.

When you worry about how to do step ten and you are still at step one, not only does it make step ten harder, it makes where you are harder too. Worry spreads through time and ends up sabotaging what you are doing right now.

Louise wanted to sculpt a series of pots for an exhibition, yet every time she sat down to sculpt she started worrying about steps well ahead of what she was trying to do. How she would market her work? How she would approach a gallery? How she would sell her pieces?

These things matter, but only when that is the stage she is at. Later, when Louise can take action and do something about them. Later, when she actually has a sculpture to sell.

Worrying now does not help Louise. It sabotages what she is doing. Worrying about how to sell the sculpture stops her being able to confidently sculpt it.

When your mind slips to your end goal, pull your attention back to what you are doing now. If you feel yourself starting to worry about how you will put all the pieces together, place your attention on just the piece in front of you now. I call this 'spot focus': remove all other thoughts from you mind and ask yourself, 'Right now, what is in front of me that I *can* do?'

Doing a pursuit is a bit like doing a puzzle. Once you put down the first few pieces the next pieces get easier. Once you put the first piece down you have something to work with. Each piece helps reveal the next. Each piece makes the next easier both to choose and to place.

Put down the pieces of the puzzle that you are able to right now and keep your attention where you are right now. This is how you sustain your confidence to put all the pieces down.

Do not worry if you do not know where all the pieces of the puzzle go or how they fit together.

Just find where the piece in your hand right now should go. Make your motto this: keep your mind where you physically are.

If your mind wanders and worries, bring it back to what is physically in front of you. If you sit down to sculpt, keep your mind on your hands and the sculpture there in front of you. This is where your confidence resides. Bring your attention to what is here — what is real now. Today there is a chunk of clay in front of you, waiting for you sculpt.

Ask yourself:

When has keeping your eye on the goal overwhelmed you?

How will you keep your focus closer to where you are right now?

Confidence is a
present time feeling;
the closer you keep
your focus to what
you are doing, the
easier it is to feel
confident.

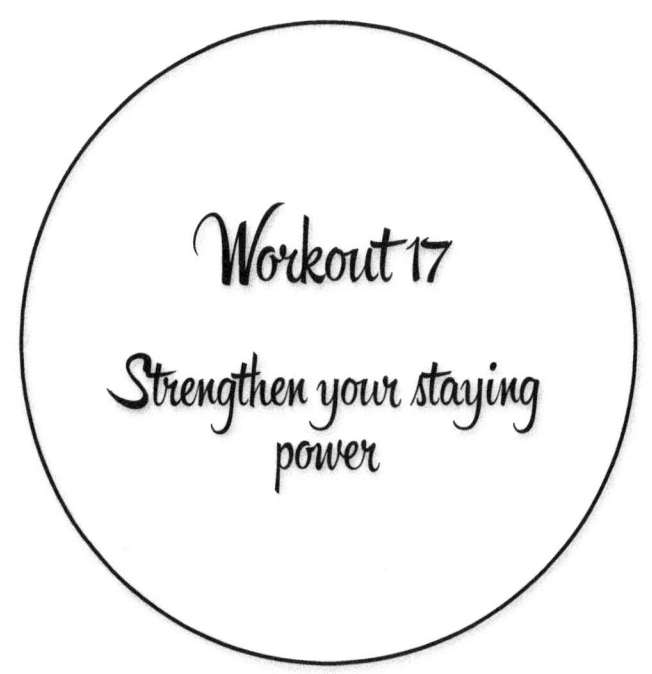

Workout 17

Strengthen your staying power

It's a nice thought to think that the road to what you want to do will be all smooth sailing, but thinking this way does not give you confidence. Expecting difficulty is what will give you the confidence.

This surprises most people. It sounds negative, almost defeatist. But it's not.

When we start with the expectation that along the way there will be setbacks, difficulties and a few bumps in the road, it builds our endurance. It does this in a few different ways.

Expecting some difficulties makes us question our staying power. It makes us more likely to nurture our endurance, too. It makes us more prepared for what's ahead and more willing to pick ourselves back up and keep going. And most of all, it makes us rally up inside ourselves and realise it's *only* worth starting *if we are willing* to endure the odd setback and have some staying power.

Starting with the expectation that there may be a few setbacks stops us personalising those setbacks if they do happen. It helps us see setbacks as a normal part of any journey and stops us blaming ourselves.

When Carol set out to change careers she thought it would be easy. She wasn't prepared when she started to receive one rejection letter after another. She immediately turned on herself with self-blame saying comments like, 'I am useless, I have no talent, I don't have what it takes.'

Carol was too quick to blame herself. She started crushing her own confidence by blaming who she was for what had happened instead of realising the path forward may be bumpy, despite who she was and what she did.

There is nothing personal about setbacks. Sometimes things don't go to plan, sometimes we get a no instead of a yes, and sometimes we don't get what we want. Setbacks happen for a whole host of reasons that usually have nothing to do with who we are.

They happen to everyone. They happen when we are talented and experienced and they happen when we are beginners.

When we accept setbacks as a normal and expected part of any endeavour, it helps us handle the setbacks with more confidence. It helps us keep our judging-self quiet and just focus on navigating the setbacks instead of blaming ourselves for them.

When we expect setbacks, it stops us overreacting to the first difficulty that comes our way. It stops us giving up too early and giving up just because one thing has gone wrong. Most of all, it helps us stay confident about ourselves and what we are doing, despite the setback.

If you are about to drive down a dirt road in your car and you see a sign that says, 'Passable, but there are bumps ahead' you will proceed in a totally different way than if you didn't know there were potholes and bumps along the road.

You respond differently. When you expect to encounter bumps, you are not surprised when you see them. You don't complain or panic. You certainly don't consider doing a u-turn at the first pothole you encounter.

You drive differently too. You are on the lookout. You are prepared that you might have to make some adjustments to navigate what is ahead.

Awaken your endurance. Expect that the road you are about to travel down will have bumps on it. Start your pursuit as if there is a sign in front of you saying, 'Passable, but there are bumps ahead.'

Accept that there will be difficulties and setbacks before starting, not when you are in the middle of them.

Ask yourself now before you even start how many bumps you can endure. Ask yourself before you start how many setbacks you are prepared to deal with and still keep going.

You don't want to be asking yourself for the first time whether you will keep going when you have a rejection letter in your hand. You will be feeling too vulnerable and dejected. You need to establish it before you send your application letter.

Knowing you are prepared to endure setbacks before you encounter them gives you sticking power right from the start. It helps you respond with confidence to whatever comes your way.

Having endurance is not something fixed. It is a choice best made right at the start. When you decide you can endure ten, twenty or even fifty rejections, then when the first one comes, you won't even ask the question *will I keep going?* You'll just keep going.

When you knock and nobody opens the door, it won't occur to you to give up. You'll knock on the door again. You'll knock in different ways and on different doors. You will keep going.

Ask yourself:

How many setbacks are you prepared to deal with and still keep going?

How will you nurture your staying power?

Start your
pursuit as if
there is a sign
in front of you
saying, 'Passable,
but there are
bumps ahead'.

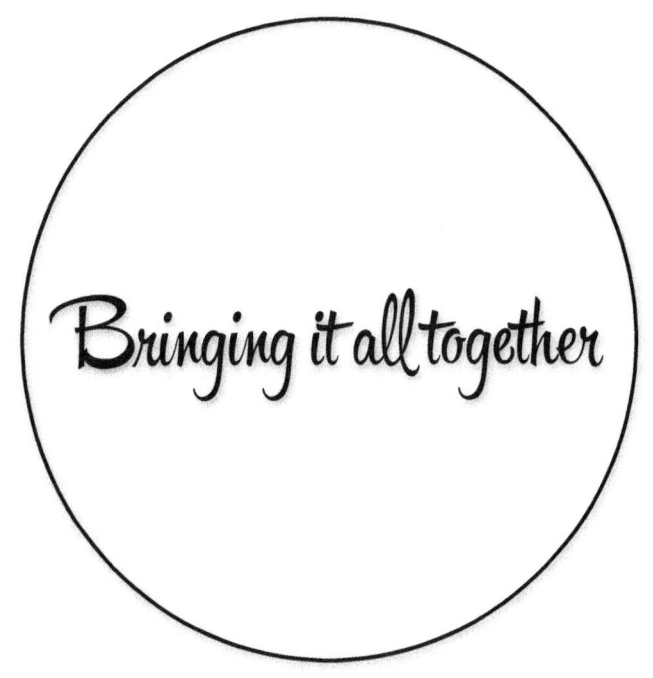

Bringing it all together

Confidence is not something you work on once and then can forget all about. Confidence needs ongoing nourishing and nurturing to stay strong and intact.

Sometimes after weeks of feeling great and progressing well with your pursuit, you can wake up and momentarily lose all confidence in what you are doing. That's because confidence is not something that is solid and fixed. Even when you have worked on boosting your confidence, from time to time your confidence will falter. Do not worry if it does. Lapses in confidence are normal and they happen to everyone.

The problem is not the lapse in confidence; the problem is what we do when we have a lapse in confidence. Lapses are not a problem if we stay calm. But most of us don't stay calm. We panic. Not only do we have a lapse in confidence; we make it doubly bad by having a crisis about our lapse in confidence.

What catches us out most is the suddenness in which this lapse in confidence can happen. It seems to slip away quickly and often without an obvious reason, yet there is always a trigger.

Lapses in confidence are triggered by many factors, including our mood, our thoughts or our attitudes. Sometimes the lapse is triggered by physical factors: we might be behind on sleep or perhaps are trying to do too much. Other times the lapses may be triggered by external factors; a comment from someone, a negative evaluation or not getting the results we were expecting.

The next time you have a lapse in confidence remind yourself that the calmer you are about your lapse in confidence the quicker you will move through it. Acknowledge it as a fact, not a concern. Say to yourself, 'Right now I'm not feeling confident' in the same calm way you would say, 'Right now I'm not feeling hungry.'

Despite your lack of confidence, still take action. Confidence does not come back by waiting, it returns by taking action. Despite how you feel, take action. Return to a corner of your work that is familiar, a step that is known or a part of your project that you know how to do easily.

See yourself as 'a confident person having a lapse in confidence' rather than 'someone who lacks confidence'. Even if you have twenty lapses of confidence every day, still position confidence as your core and your foundation.

Speak as though it is temporary. Act like it is temporary. This will help you retain a sense of hope that things will change. That's because every next moment holds all sorts of different possibilities. Confident possibilities.

Confidence is constructed. Each day we get to rebuild it through the actions we take and choices we make.

Think of your confidence as a fire that you want to keep alight. To keep the fire burning you will have to tend to it from time to time. You have to stoke it.

Throughout life there will be times when you need to stoke your confidence. There will be pivotal moments when you need to be more alert. In the midst of any change — when you start something new or end something familiar — your confidence will almost always be more fragile.

Don't wait to rekindle your confidence when all you are left with is embers. Nourish it and nurture your confidence routinely. Do it at the start of anything new and at every step along the way. Make caring for your confidence part of how you live.

You have so much more potential, talent and happiness inside you than you can imagine. It's time to stop holding back and awaken that part in you that is ready to take your next step.

Remember confidence does not come from one big thing. For most of us our confidence grows from the sum of all the little positive things we do and together they begin to transform how we feel and what we do.

Enjoy your journey and all the wonderful things that feeling confident will allow you to do.

Michelle

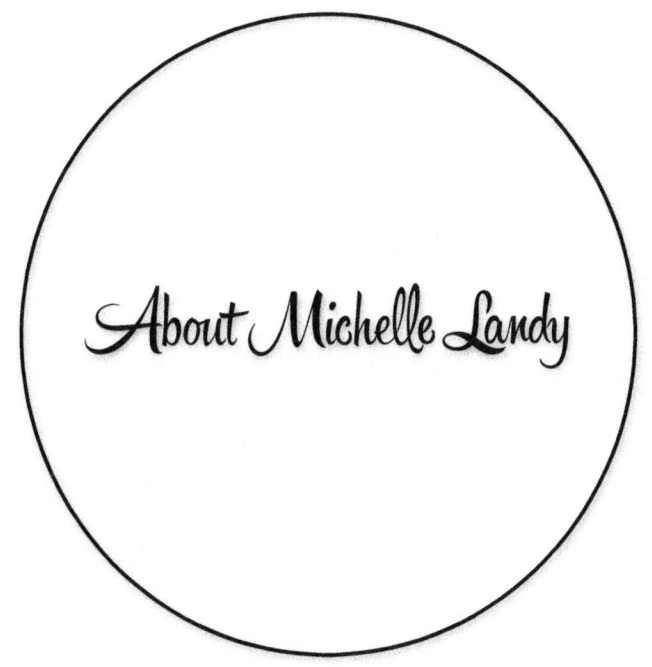

About Michelle Landy

Michelle Landy is a presenter, author and coach. She inspires people around the world with her messages of self-belief and positive change.

She is founder of the coaching program, 'The Confidence Workout', from which this book has been written, helping people turn their hesitation and self-doubt into confidence and action.

Since graduating from university with a B.A. with a focus on behavioural science and a Post

Graduate degree in Business with a focus on performance and training, Michelle has continued her own research into achieving positive change. She is a master NLP practitioner, a coach and a qualified facilitator.

Michelle is an honorary lecturer at the University of Technology, Sydney, helping people advance their careers.

The media regularly interview Michelle for her expert opinion on a wide range of subjects including achieving goals, career tips, building confidence and raising children with self-esteem.

Michelle is married with three gorgeous children.

Contact Michelle Landy

To book Michelle Landy for your next event email: info@michellelandy.com

To find out more about Michelle Landy go to: www.michellelandy.com

To let Michelle know about your confidence breakthroughs: info@michellelandy.com